When Our Mom had Cancer

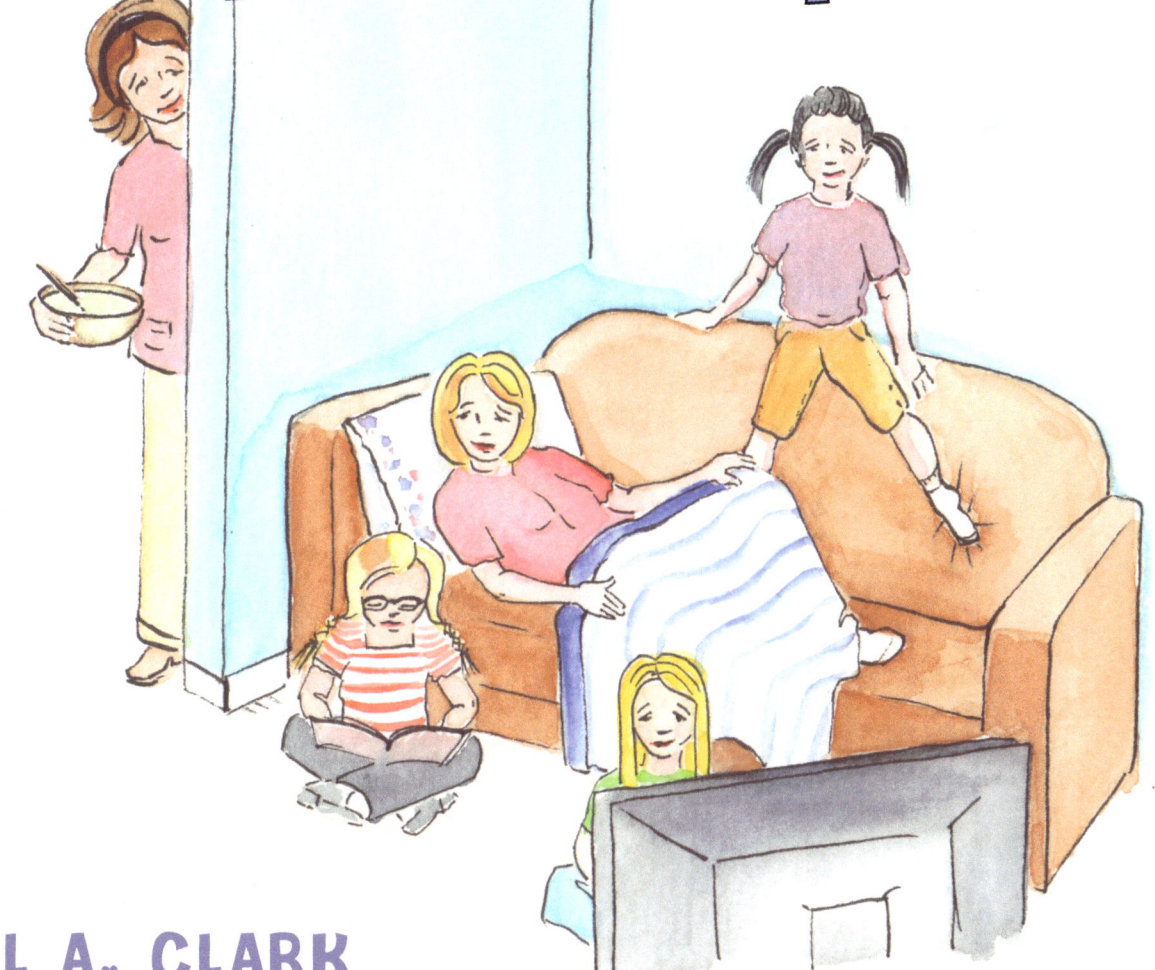

CAROL A. CLARK

ILLUSTRATED BY MARY DOLAN

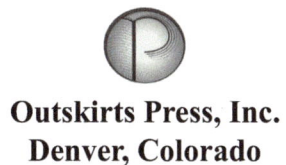

Outskirts Press, Inc.
Denver, Colorado

To my fantastic husband, Mike, who understands and puts up with me after all these years.

To my three daughters, Sara, Kelly and Emily who make me proud every single day. I am so lucky to be your mom.

And, to my friend, Kathy, who helped me through treatment and encouraged me to write a book.

When Our Mom had Cancer
All Rights Reserved.
Copyright © 2010 Carol A. Clark
v3.0

Illustrated by Mary Dolan.

Outskirts Press, Inc.
http://www.outskirtspress.com

ISBN: 978-1-4327-5129-6

Library of Congress Control Number: 2009942814

Outskirts Press and the "OP" logo are trademarks belonging to Outskirts Press, Inc.

PRINTED IN THE UNITED STATES OF AMERICA

This Book Belongs to:

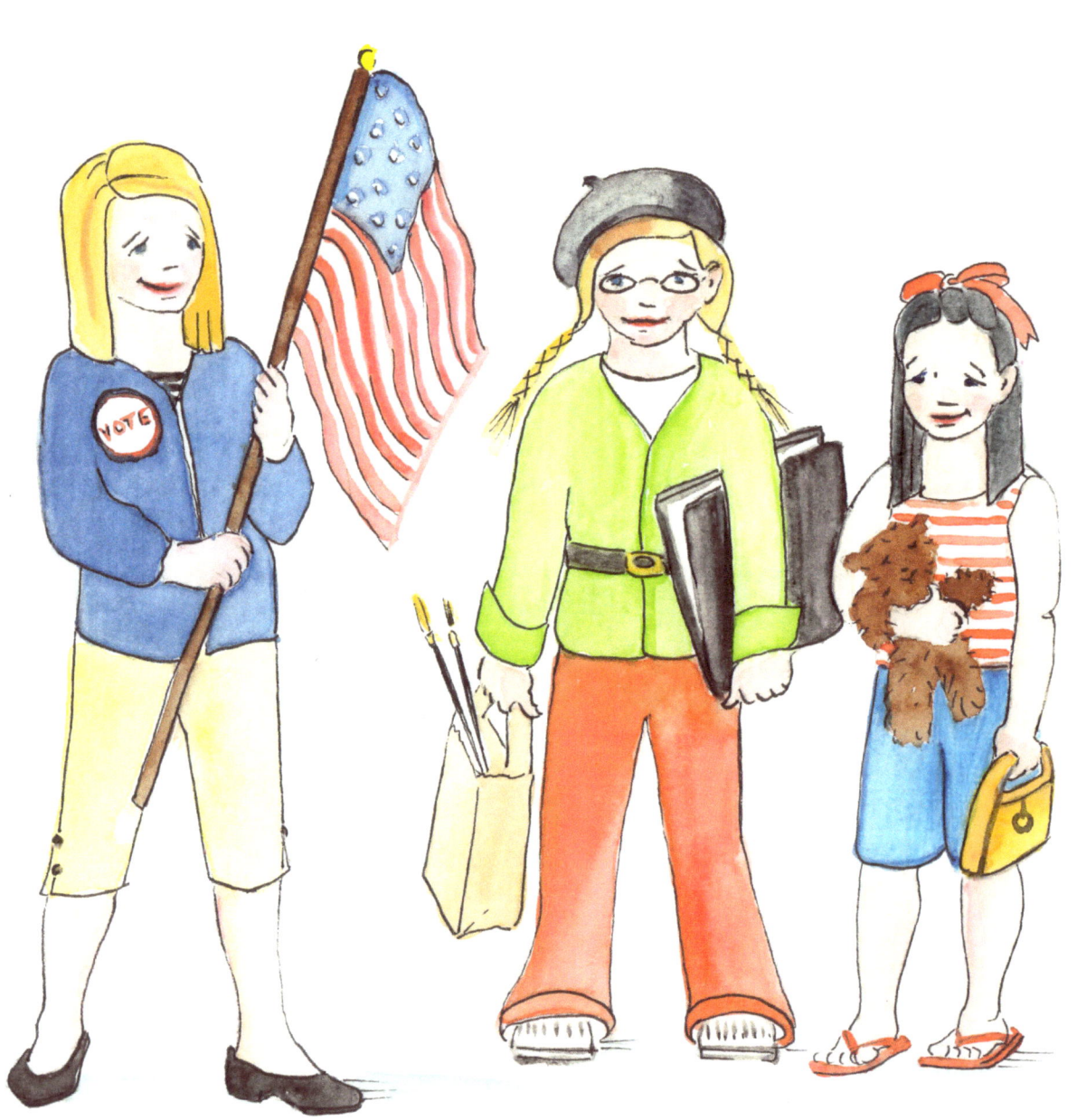

My name is Sara. I am the oldest kid in our family. Someday I want to be President.

My name is Kelly. I am the middle kid and I love art.

My name is Emily. Some people call me the baby of the family but I don't really like that.

One day our Mommy and Daddy told us that we needed to have a talk.

Sara thought we were getting a puppy.

Kelly thought we were going on a trip.

Emily thought we were getting a present.

None of our guesses were right. Instead, Mommy and Daddy told us that Mom had something called cancer. We didn't really know what that was but we could tell it was not something fun like a puppy, a trip, or a present.

Mommy said that sometimes people's cells go crazy and make them sick. That's what happened to her. She explained that she would have an operation and then the doctor would give her really strong medicine to help kill the bad cancer cells. Some of the medicine might make Mommy seem sick. We were scared and we cried a little bit. Mommy said that she would be going to the hospital where we were born. That made us feel a little better.

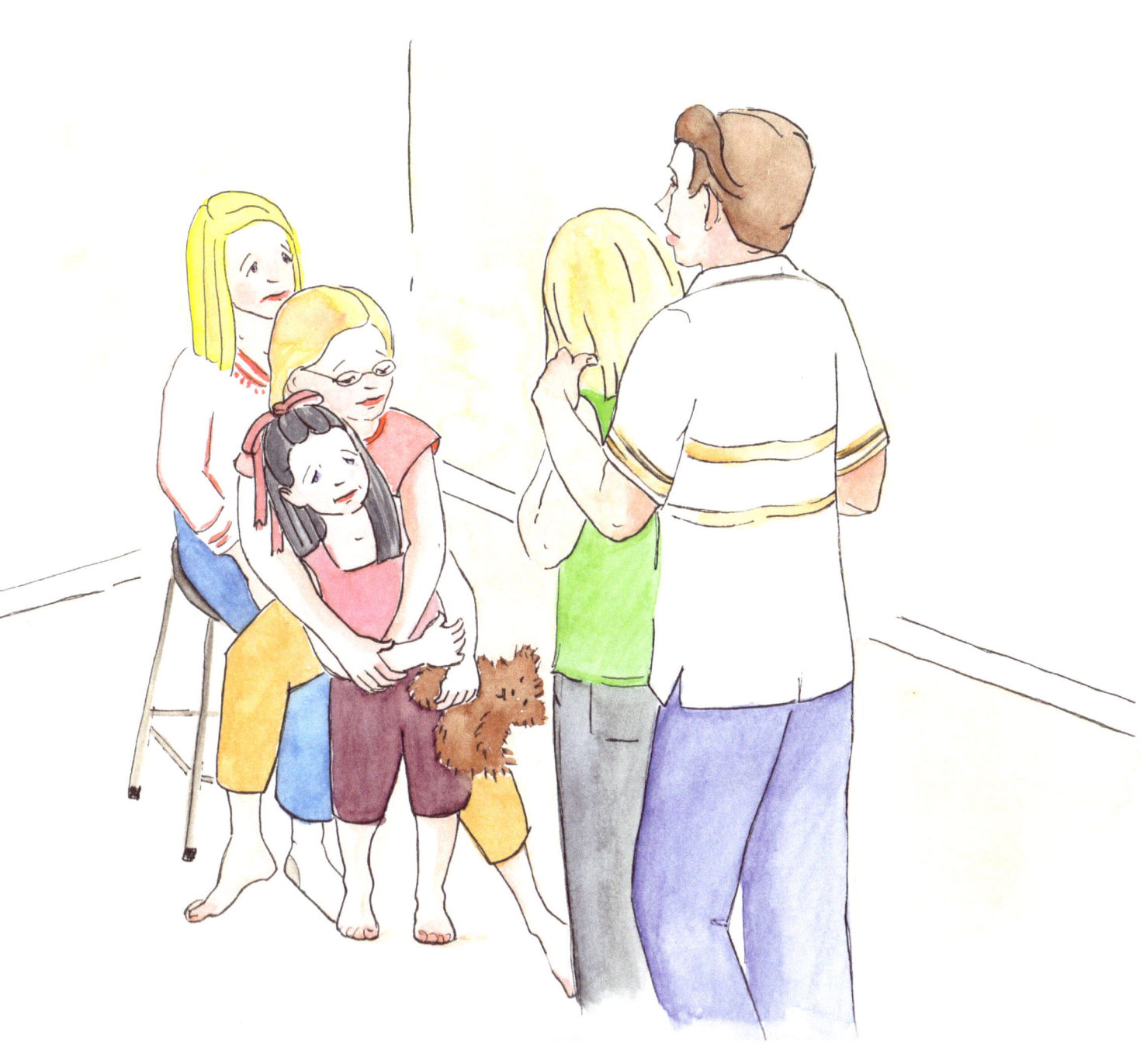

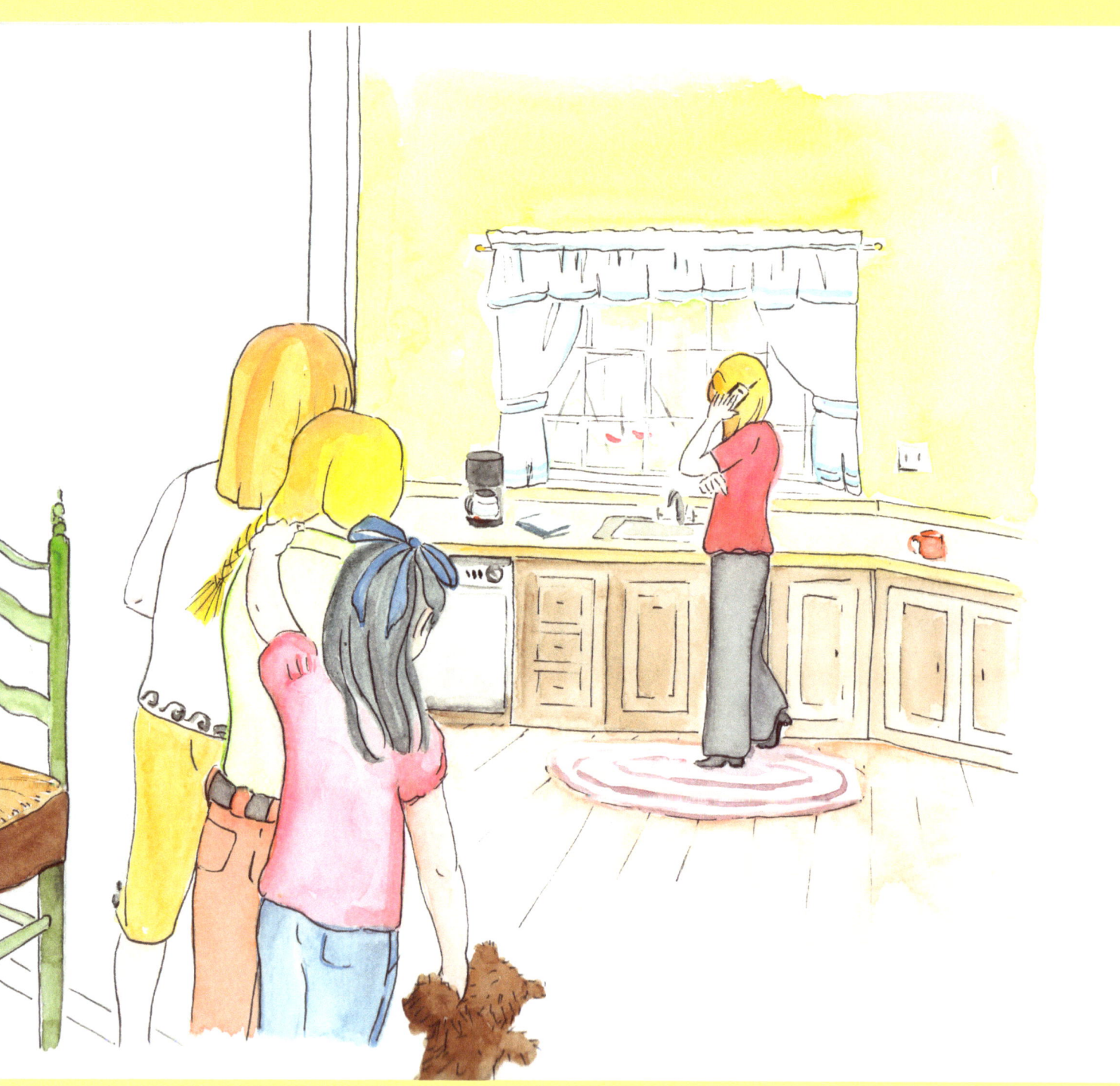

We could tell Mommy was worried because she talked on the phone. We think that talking on the phone must have made Mommy feel better because she did it a lot.

Soon it was time for Mommy's operation. She left the house early in the morning. We thought about her all day.

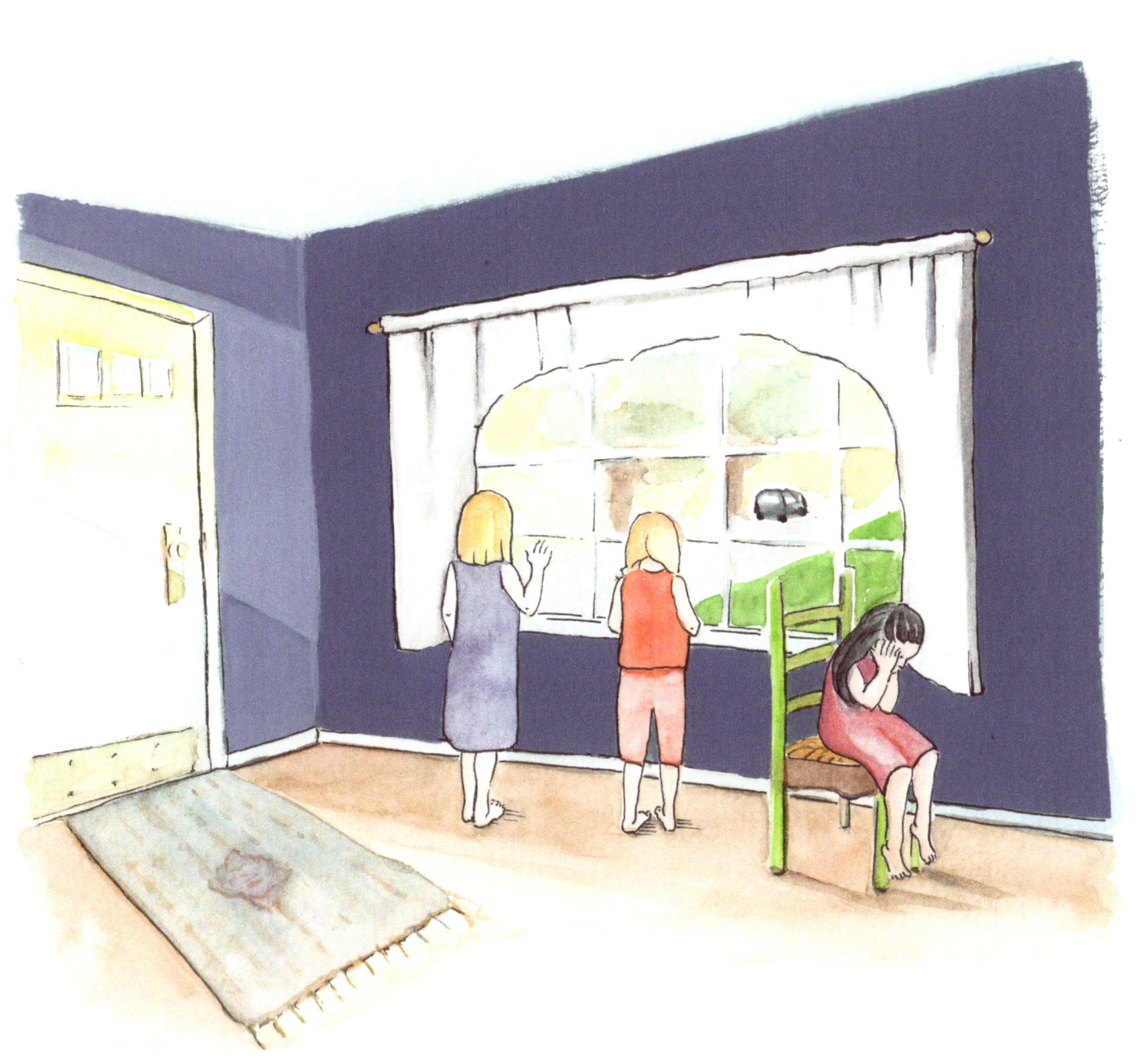

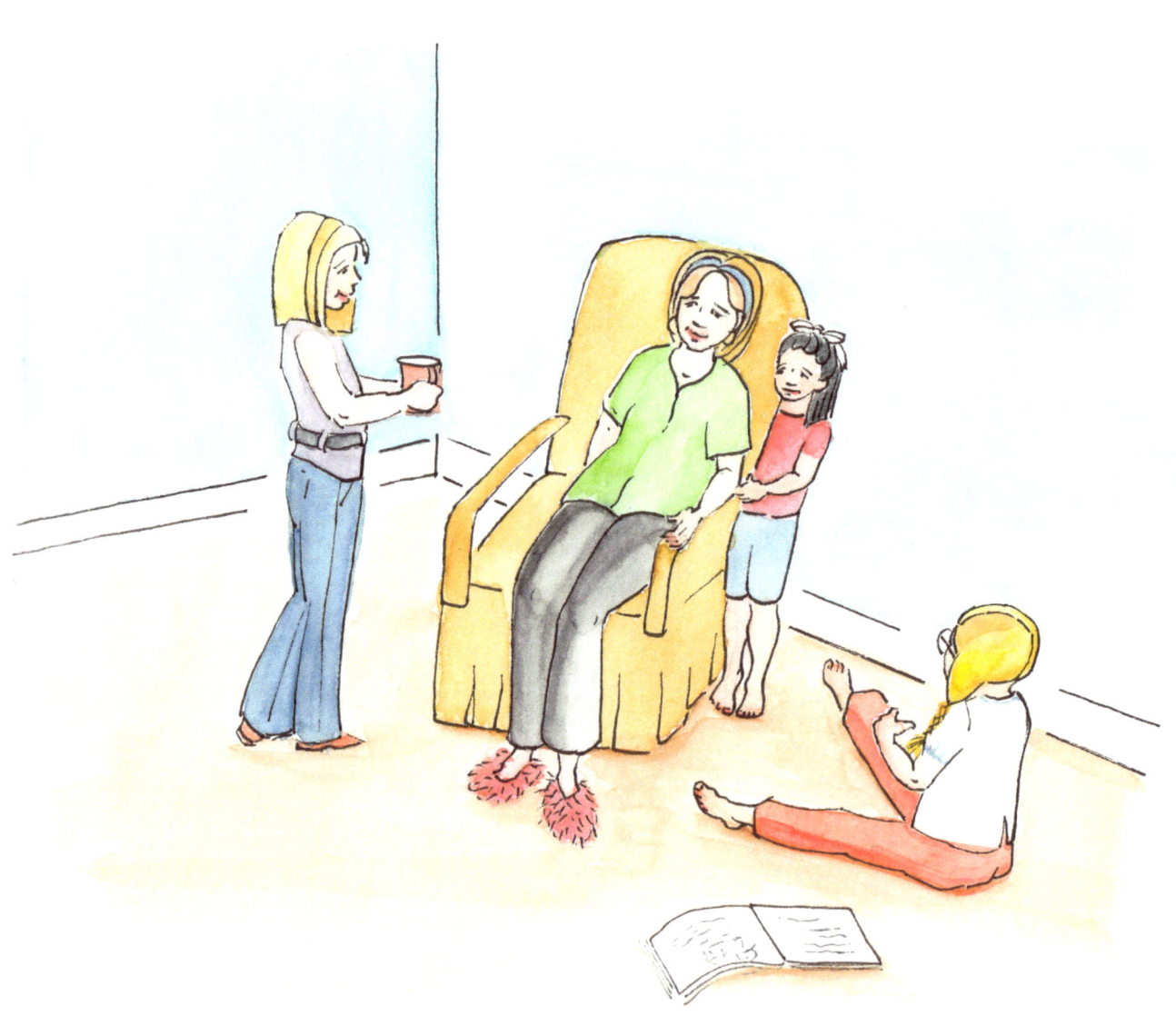

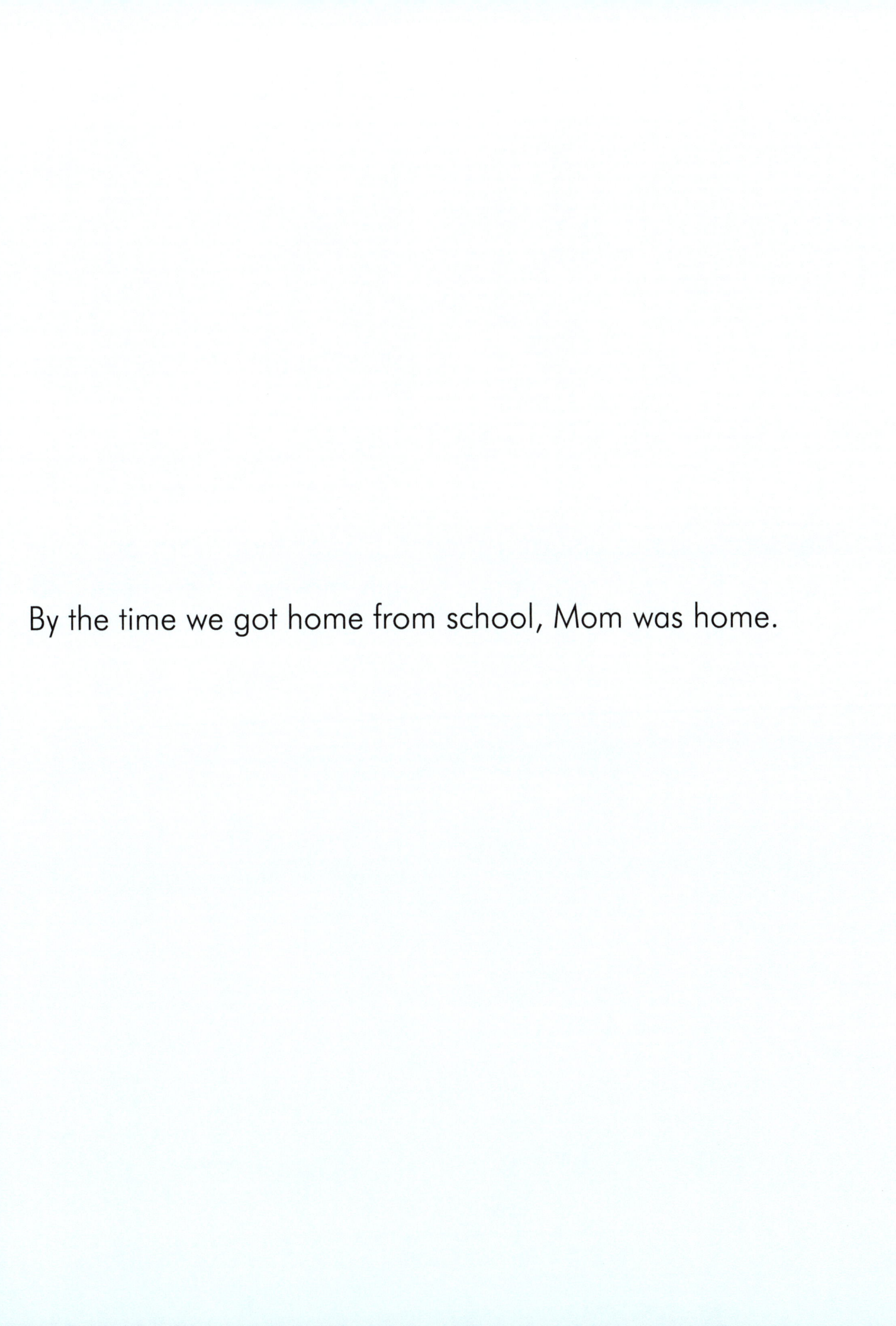

By the time we got home from school, Mom was home.

She slept a lot at first and moved slower than normal. Our Mommy, like most mommies, usually moves fast so it seemed a little strange to us.

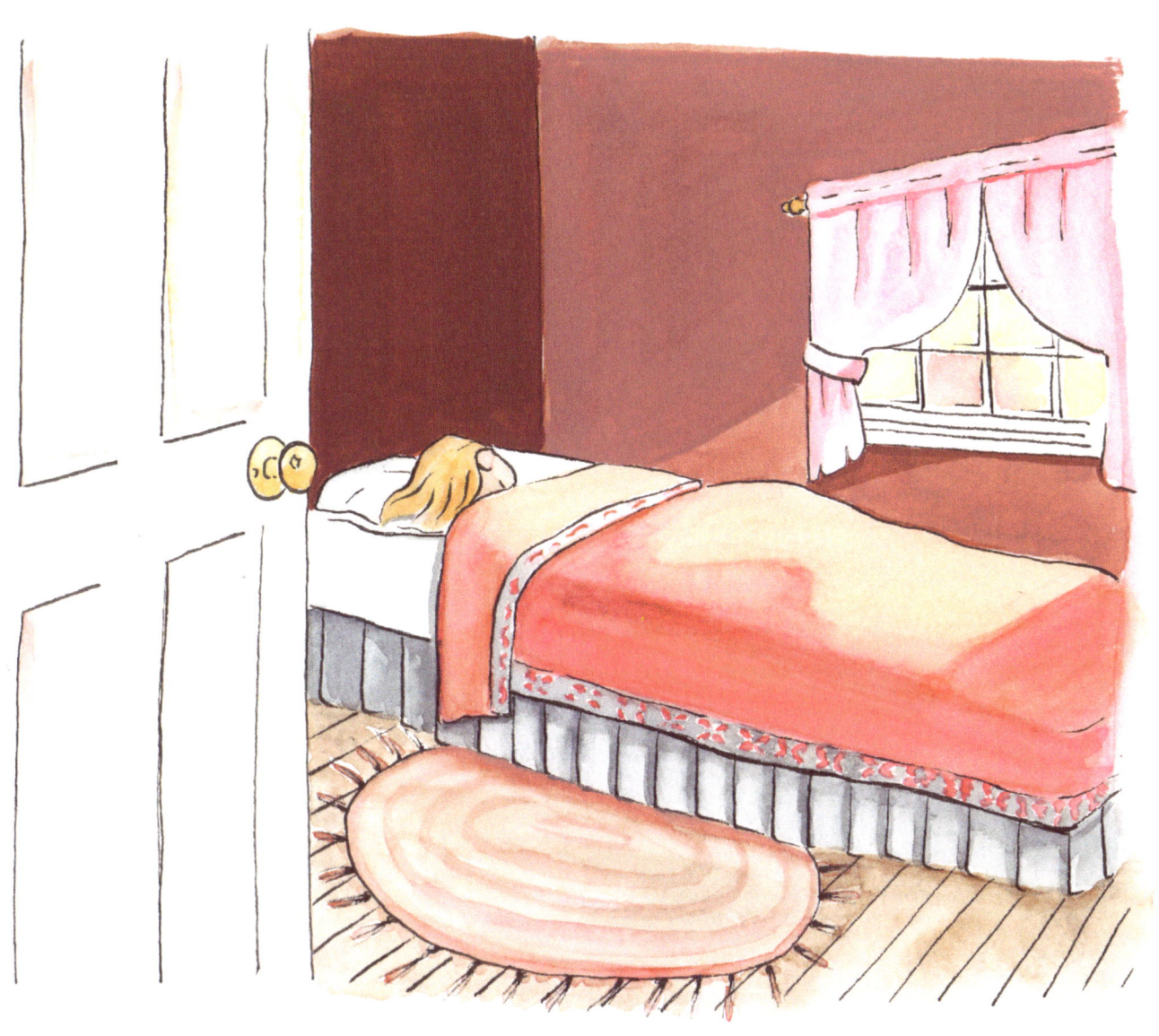

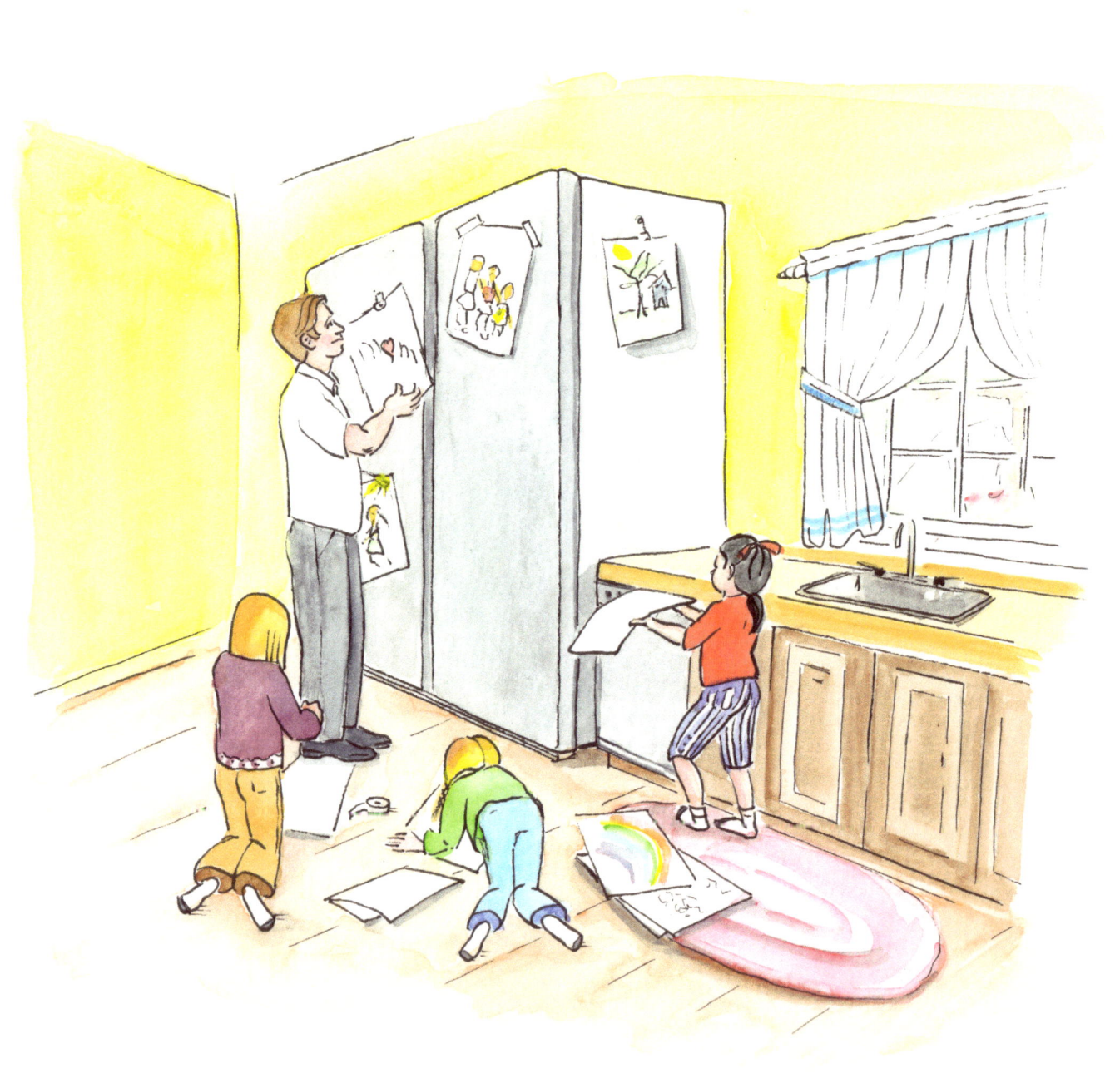

Daddy stayed home from work for a few days so that part was fun. We drew lots of get well pictures for Mom. She said they made her feel tons better. It made us feel better too.

Next, Mommy explained that even though the cancer was taken out by the doctor, there could still be some small bits of cancer left that the doctor could not see.

One way to kill cancer is to have a kind of medicine, called chemotherapy. She told us it is sort of like when you eat a cookie and you drop the crumbs. The whole cookie is gone but you still need to clean up the crumbs. That was the job of chemotherapy. Most people call it chemo for short.

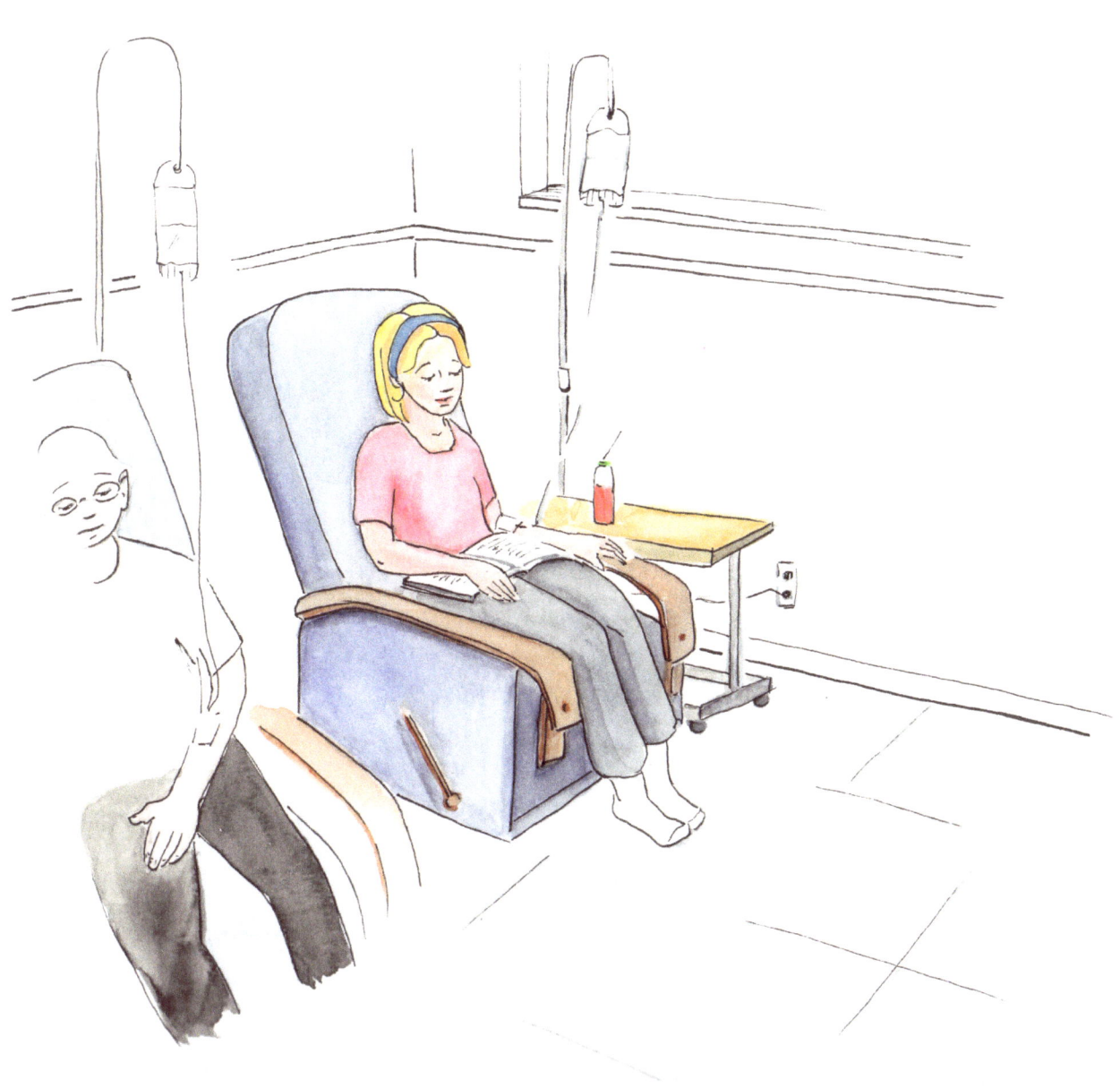

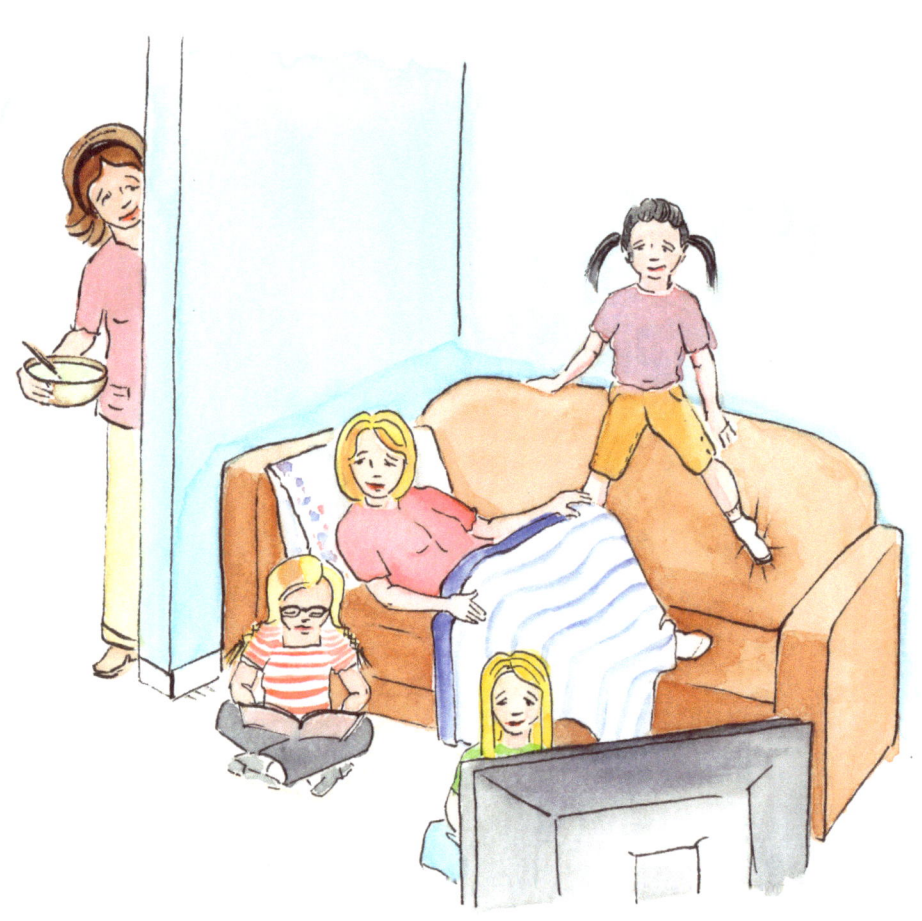

The chemo made Mommy feel yucky but she was still our Mom and she still took care of us.

When she didn't feel well she would lay on the couch and watch cartoons with us. We liked that part. Sometimes we read stories to her. She liked that. There were some things that were different. Sometimes people would bring us food for dinner.

Other times we would go to a friend's house. And some of the time our grandparents would come to take care of us while Mommy was resting or visiting the doctor. It was fun eating new foods, playing with friends, and seeing relatives.

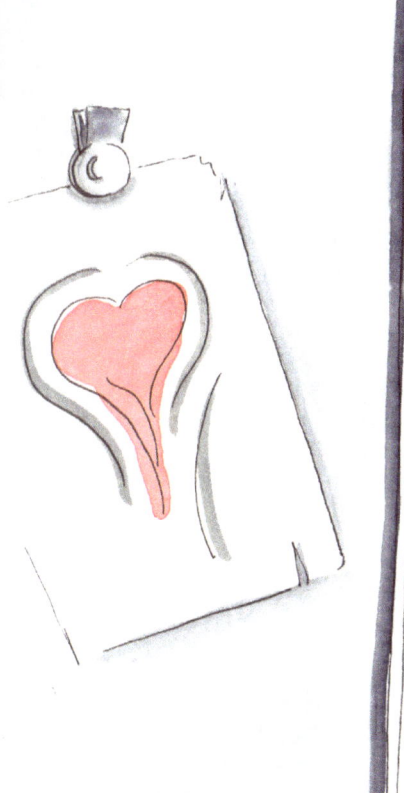

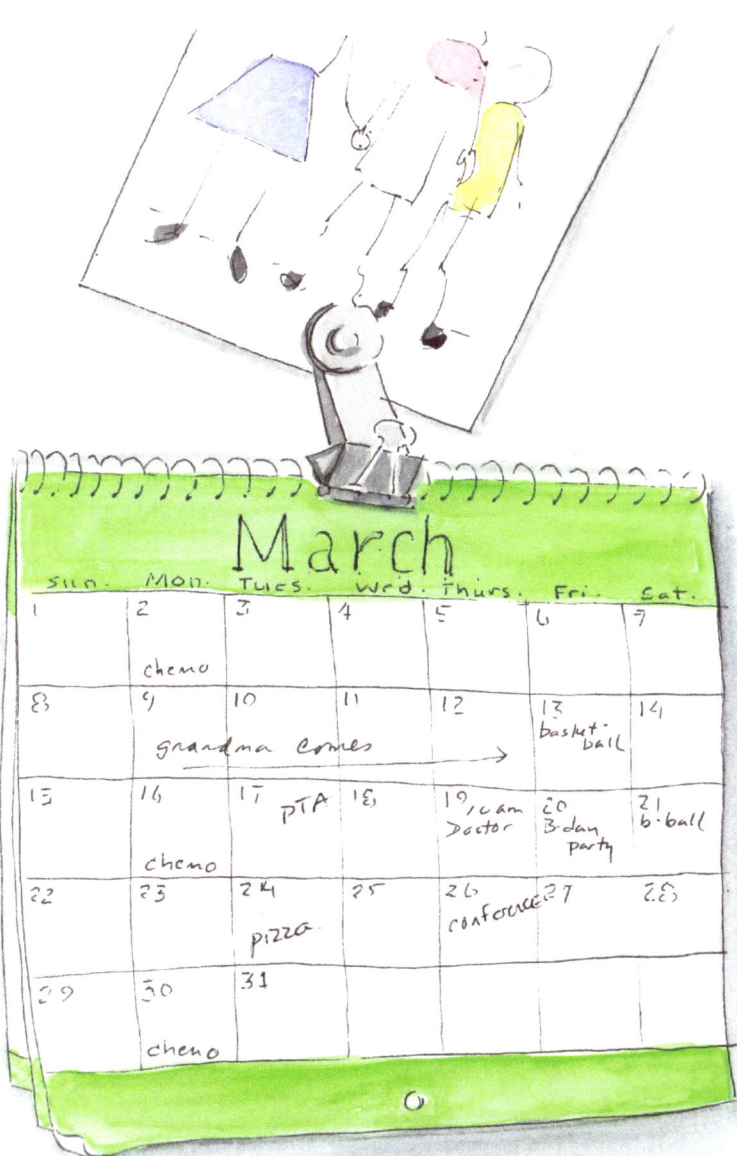

March

Sun.	Mon.	Tues.	Wed.	Thurs.	Fri.	Sat.
1	2 chemo	3	4	5	6	7
8	9	10 grandma comes	11	12	13 basket-ball	14
15	16 chemo	17 PTA	18	19 I am Doctor	20 B-day party	21 b-ball
22	23	24 pizza	25	26 conference	27	28
29	30 chemo	31				

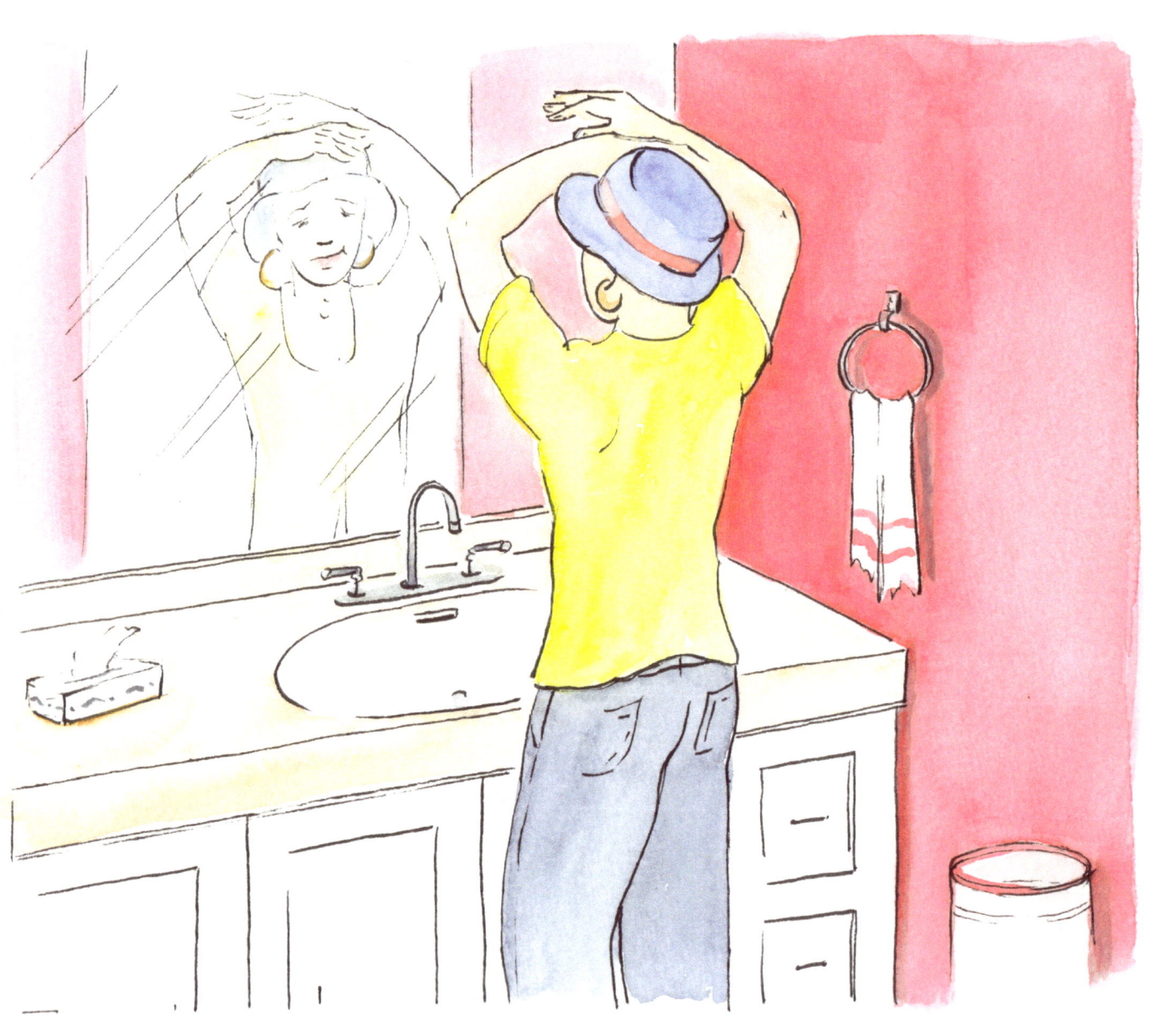

The worst part of chemo was when Mommy's hair fell out. We knew that it was going to happen because Mommy told us ahead of time.

After a while we got used to it and Mommy was still Mommy.

She was just Mommy with a hat.

She still played with us as usual, helped us with our homework, read stories to us, and snuggled with us.

Mommy had to have chemo for a bunch of months and we thought it would take forever, but before we knew it, she was done with it. She was glad to be finished and we were glad too.

Soon Mommy's hair began to grow back. She was still tired and slept more than usual but it didn't take long for Mommy to be regular Mommy again.

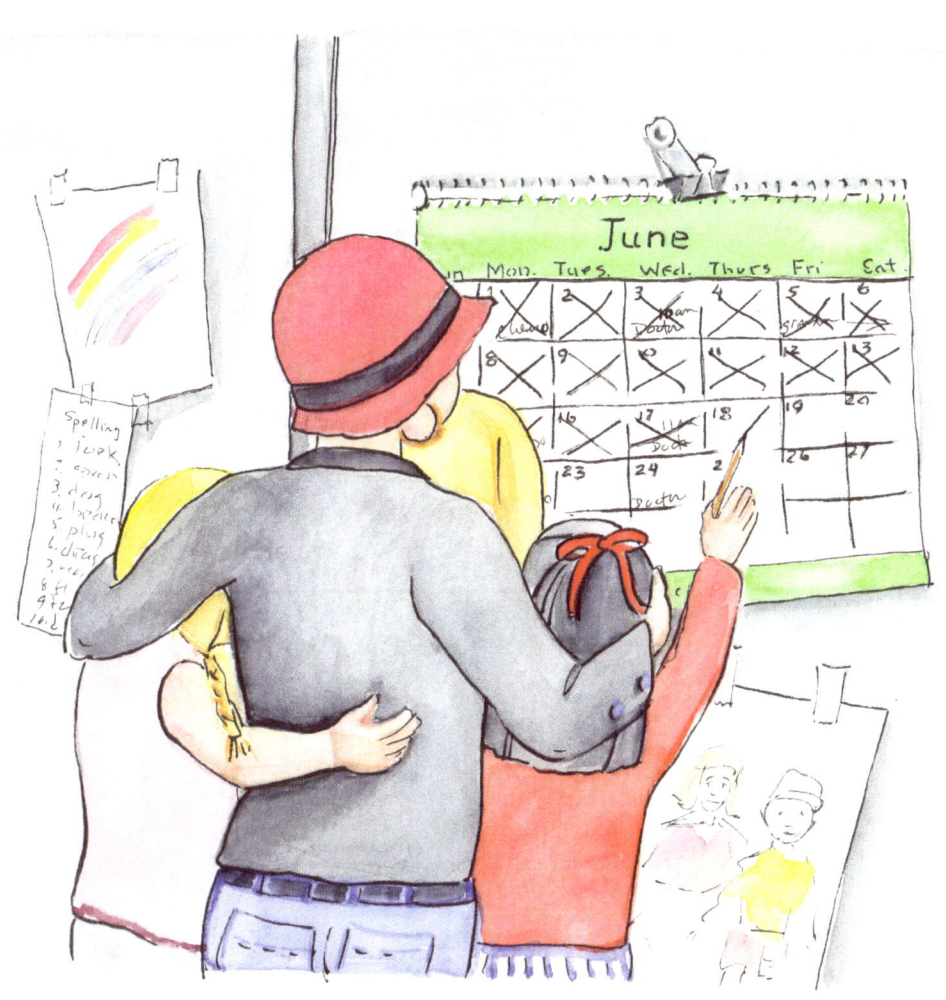

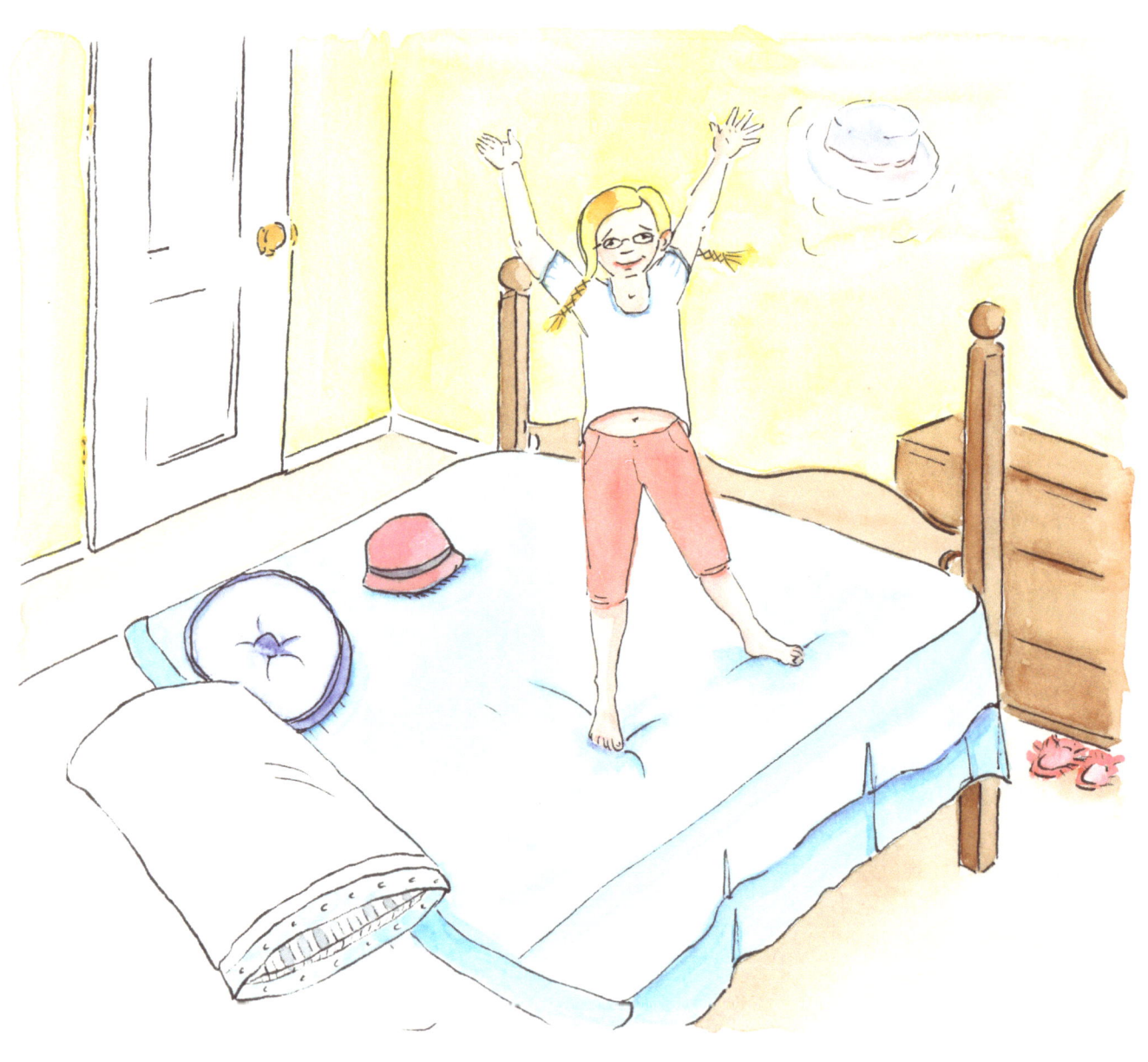

Mommy says that she is proud of the way we handled everything.
We are proud of her too.

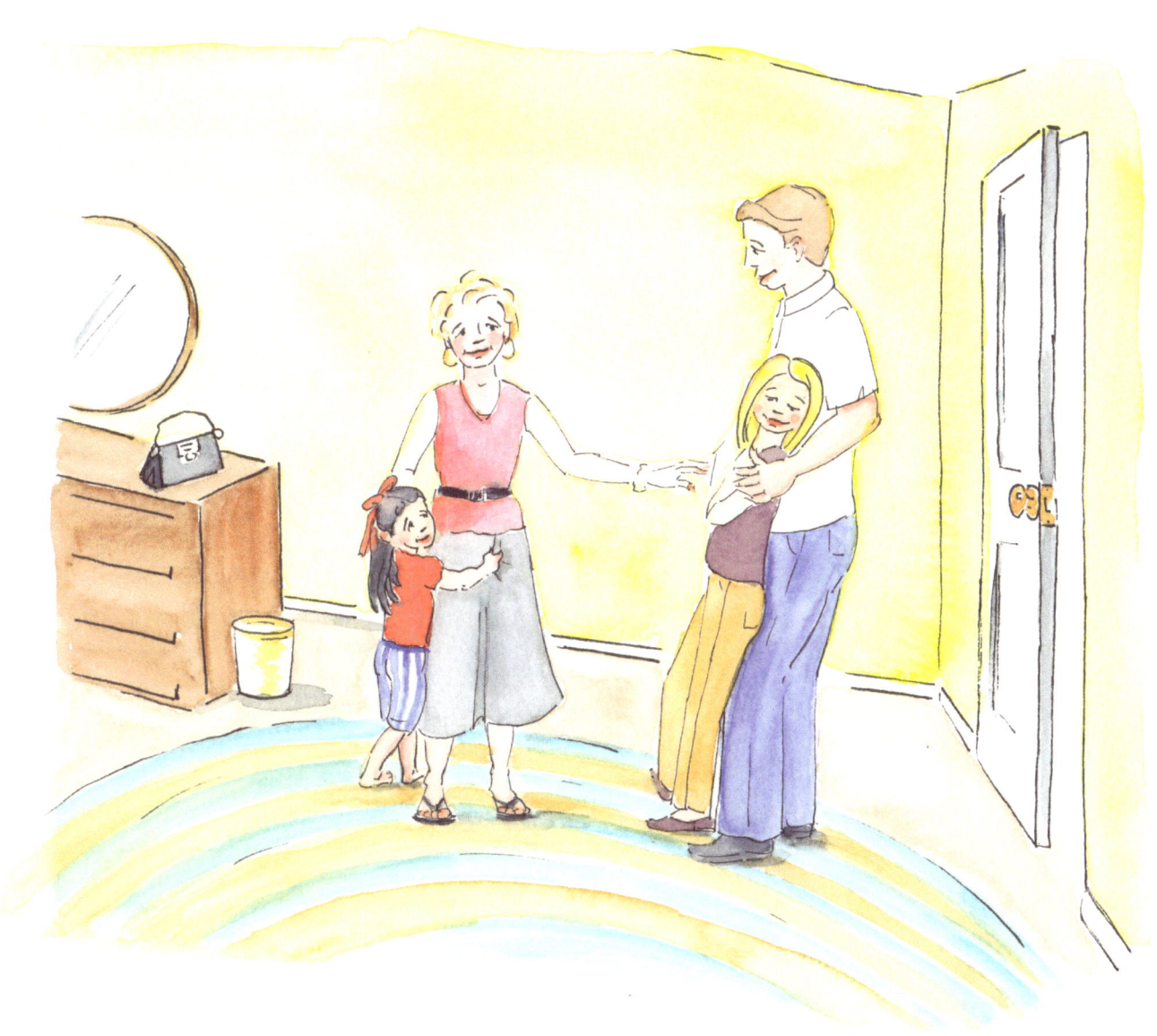

Now things are back to normal. Sara still wants to be President, Kelly still loves art, and Emily still doesn't like to be called the baby of the family.